JUICING RECIPES

From Fitlife.TV Star Drew Canole

FOR VITALITY AND HEALTH

By DREW CANOLE

Copyright 2012 FitLife TV, LLC

ISBN-13: 978-1481954266

MIH Publishing

BRAND NEW BOOK FROM AUTHOR

DREW CANOLE!

On SALE Now On Amazon.com!

"Train Your Taste To Trim Your Waist:

**A Simple Method To
Love The Food That Loves You Back"**

http://trainyourtaste.com/juicingrecipes

This groundbreaking new book from Drew Canole is on sale now, exclusively at Amazon.

Revealing a simple, step-by-step method that anyone can use, to finally flip the switch and love the food that loves you back!

This is the follow up book to "Juicing Recipes" that you're reading right now.

Table of Contents

***

A Juice-fueled Journey

My sincerest hope is that this book changes your life. No matter what your overall health goal is, juicing has the potential to reshape not only your physical landscape but also your internal workings as well. Ever hear of the expression, "Green on the inside, clean on the inside?"

Simply drinking just a few glasses a day will supply the essential vitamins and minerals your body needs.

Some major benefits are:

They are easy to make, and take just minutes to prepare.

They are made in your own kitchen, so you know exactly what's in them.

They supply you with massive amounts of nutrients that your body needs.

You will feel the power of raw energy once the juice hits your blood stream.

Juices leave you energized all day.

One of the foremost reasons I was able to go from 17 percent body fat down to sub-7 percent was because of juicing. Not *that* kind of juicing—I'm talking straight-up, 100 percent pure "green" veggie juice. And maybe an occasional apple or other fruit for taste.

I was first turned on to juicing by my good friend William Ripley. He told me the devastating tale of his heroic father who had recently suffered a heart attack. The doctors had given him a very short time to live—unless he were to make some pretty radical changes immediately. At the time, his father was severely overweight, his testosterone was at an

1

all-time low, and he had very little, if any, energy whatsoever. What's sad is that 70 percent of the population suffers in the same way as Mr. Ripley.

Determined to get better, Mr. Ripley set out to find a solution to his failing health problem. He visited multiple doctors, and tried various homeopathic remedies along with an expansive array of other methods for healing. He was at a friend's house when he shared his bad news and explained his situation to her. He asked her for advice, with an, "I'll do whatever it takes—I'm about to die" look on his face.

Within a moment she pulled out a juicer from her small pantry and gathered veggies from the fridge. As she washed the vegetables, Mr. Ripley started to chuckle.

"What are we going to do with *those*?" he asked.

FACT: Most people in America are now getting two or less servings of vegetables a day when they should be getting seven to ten.

Mr. Ripley's friend's response was simple. "We are going to juice them."

Mr. Ripley was unfamiliar with the concept of juicing vegetables, but he was desperate and ready to do whatever it would take. Simply put: he was running out of time. Every heartbeat was another gift from God. Each thump reminded him of all the abuse he had laid on it, including years of poor sleeping habits and a highly toxic diet. Mr. Ripley was open for a change that day.

The juice his friend made for him consisted of a couple of carrots, a cucumber, and some ginger. She handed the cup to him and he grimaced. He had always had a disdain for the taste of carrots and had never even tasted raw ginger. But he put the glass up to his lips and took his first sip.

"This stuff tastes amazing!"

She smiled and reflected on how often she had seen this expression from newbie juicers.

After Mr. Ripley's first juice, and with the hope of losing weight and gaining health, he became a juicing addict. Not only did he start juicing three times a day, he convinced all of his neighbors to juice. They were hesitant to take him up on his invitations but they decided to out of respect and support, since they wanted to keep their friend around.

Months went by and Mr. Ripley—remaining faithful to his new love of juicing—felt more energy coursing through his veins and . dropped the excessive weight like he had the metabolism of a pre-pubescent adolescent.

Eventually the medication prescribed by his cardiologist started giving him problems. He explained to his doctor that it was causing vomiting and convulsing. The doctor quickly responded by running tests. A few hours later, the doctor came back in with results. It seemed that Mr. Ripley's immune system had strengthened so much that it had formed a "block" against the medicine.

His doctor wanted to increase the dosage of the medicine, but Mr. Ripley knew that he no longer needed it and knew that it wasn't the medicine that was improving his health and keeping him alive. It was the juice!

He had to get the secret out!

And thankfully he did.

Inspiration Strikes

After his eldest son William shared his father's heart-wrenching story, I realized that I had to get a juicer—ASAP! This would end up being the best investment for my health that I'd ever make.

At the time, I had lots of energy but was constantly searching for the nearest coffee shop for my caffeine fix. I was in good physical shape but nowhere near where I wanted to be. I would often work out twice a day, sometimes for more than three hours a day. Regardless, I just couldn't lose what looked like baby fat surrounding my abdominal region and my little chipmunk face.

Sound familiar?

Like many people, I was severely dehydrated and didn't even know it. Often I would mistake my dehydration for hunger, which forced me into overeating. For years this went on, and instead of drinking nourishing liquids I would overeat pizza and other life-draining foods. This is the story of most of the population. We are "the dehydrated nation" and also the most overweight. Do you think there is a connection?

There is—a big one!

As a culture we load up on soda, coffee, tea, alcohol, and other beverages that are not good for our physical well-being. One 20-ounce bottle of Coke has the equivalent of 16 packets of sugar in it, yet we wonder why America is fighting an obesity/diabetes epidemic, which is a leading cause of death in America.

It's no coincidence that the top three are diet-related. We are eating out of convenience and making unwise decisions when it comes to our long-term health. It takes the body more energy to process this fat-laden, sugar-loaded, processed, lifeless junk food, and we are giving ourselves less time to heal.

Through a rigorous juicing schedule, within three months, I started to see a six-pack starting to peek through my abs that I had never seen on myself before. This was enough to encourage the beginning of a lifelong habit.

Some of the transforming results that juicing brought to my life were:

- More energy
- More chiseled muscle
- More testosterone
- Healthier skin and hair
- Overall glow
- Greater mental acuteness
- Sexier

A HAPPIER DREW!

Would you like to have any of these things in your life? If you answered "yes," then it is time to learn about one of the greatest discoveries I've made up until this point.

Let me help you to "Juice Up Your Life!"

Why Should You Juice?

"All the smart kids are doing it."

And by "kids" I mean—when you juice, you feel younger, like a kid again. You just have to experience it for yourself; no one can fully capture what juicing can do for you until you have savored your first cup.

Since you probably don't have a glass of fresh vegetable juice in front of you now, let me explain the multitude of health benefits, regardless of your age, race, or current physical condition.

It has been said that we are what we eat, and it has been proven that a diet of fresh juice, legumes, organic fruits, and vegetables will aid you in obtaining great health. I consider myself living proof!

This book is not to be treated as a scientific research paper based on the thousands of trials and tests done on humans for decades on end. No, this book is about my own personal experience with juicing and the many others who have joined *The New Lean* revolution in order to take ownership once and for all of their physical and mental well-being.

I believe by adding fresh vegetable juice to your life you will contribute greatly to your cardiovascular health. As I sit here typing this, my resting heart rate is anywhere from 45 to 50 beats a minute. If you apply the principles in this book to your own life, you will enhance your physical performance, help your blood pressure, gain restful sleep, and increase your energy—more than you have ever imagined!

I've had many friends join me on various social media networks asking for juice recipes, and then going out and buying juicers. I receive a steady flow of emails from people who have joined the revolution and who have freed themselves from destructive habits and failing health.

Every day my friends and I are nourishing trillions of cells in our bodies with the best form of food we could ever take in. I'm not advocating that you stop eating food and drink only juice. What I am suggesting, however, is to plan out five to eight small meals a day and fresh juice in between. My small meals are basically snacks. This keeps my insulin from spiking and my metabolism revved up to the max. When your metabolism is working *for* you and not *against* you, you can stop worrying about working out so much and counting calories.

My body was laden with pounds of excessive fat and I thought the only way to rid myself of this was to work out— excessively. Boy, was I wrong. Now, I work out half as much and my body takes care of itself. Once all the toxins were removed from my system, it was much easier to lose the fat in those seemingly impossible-to-lose places.

The Benefits of Live Juice

As we all know, we are what we eat. The body needs live food to build live cells. When I say "live foods," I'm talking about foods that come directly out of the soil and are still alive. Raw foods— not cooked or processed—like beans, nuts, legumes, fruits, and my favorite . . . VEGETABLES!

When we eat live foods, our bodies consume the liquid immediately and then pass on to the lower digestive tract all of the excess. Imagine an IV of super, powerful, energy-rich foods pumped immediately into the organ of your choice, supplying all the quintessential nutrients you need for the day. The juicer does all of the work for you, so that when you drink that glass of fresh "heaven in your mouth" (that's what I call it), you feel it instantly!

The juice from the juicer is much better for you than any juice you can buy from the store, or even at the local farmer's market. When juice sits on a counter or in the fridge, it oxidizes and loses the lion's share of nutrients. Plus, juice from a juicer is not pasteurized, meaning it isn't cooked or boiled to help it stay on the shelf longer. The fresh juice is literally bursting with live energy ready to heal, pump, and energize you all day.

Many of my friends first asked me, "Why a juicer? Can't I do the same thing with a blender?" The answer, simply, is, "No." Using a blender puts pulp into your juice, which is the same thing as eating the whole thing. Your body still has to expend energy to break it down. While your body does need fiber—and I do advocate eating plenty of fresh fruits and vegetables—the juicer provides you with a cup of pure, unadulterated vitamins and minerals.

FACT: One cup of raw carrot juice contains the same amount of nutrients as four cups of diced carrots. Carrot juice tastes like a sweet dessert—without the guilt—and leaves you with energy instead of crashing from a sugar rush.

Ninety-five percent of the nourishment from fruit and vegetable juice is immediately released into the blood stream because there is nothing interfering with the processing once it hits your stomach. Before I started juicing, I would consume enough vitamins and supplements to open a pharmacy. After juicing for a while, I could tell that the vitamins would have to go because I was already supplying my body with all it needed through the juice alone! So, when you consider the costly vitamins that also take up valuable space in your cabinets, it's a no-brainer: move the veggies in and kick out the supplements.

Veggie vs. Fruit Juice

It's important to know the difference between the two.

Vegetables are much more difficult to digest. They tend to be much bulkier and break down slower in the body. When I drink green veggie juice, my mind and body reward me immediately with lasting energy and immunity.

You see, vegetables are the building blocks of life! They are responsible for providing you with strong healthy bones, tissues, muscles, and nerve support. When you consume vegetables, you can rest assured that you are getting all—or most—of the nutrients, minerals, and vitamins you need for that day.

Whole fruits are much easier to digest than vegetables and always should be taken separately. If I'm going to indulge in a fruit juice, I'll leave a window of 30 minutes to an hour before I eat or drink anything else. Most fruits—like apples, pears, and plums—contain a lot of digestive enzymes that will keep your digestive system regular. Fruits have the lion's share of the antioxidants your body requires as well.

Fruits give me radical amounts of energy before I make my way into the gym at 6:00 every morning. On occasion, I'll have a cheat day where I skip the gym and eat a bunch of not-so-good carbs, like rice or potatoes. On these days, I'll prepare by drinking fresh grapefruit juice. This helps control my insulin levels, keeping me a lean machine—even on cheat days.

Vegetable juicing is always best when you're trying to lose weight. The minerals and high-potassium content hydrate your cells and force out the sodium that causes water retention. Regularly drinking vegetable juice helps super-boost your health and remove toxins in your body.

Many of the green drinks are effective at pushing out excess water and toxins that could be causing your cells to retain fat. For example, the Mega Man Green Drink will get rid of the excess water from your cells. The Mega Man consists of kale, spinach, celery, lemon, dandelion greens, cucumber, and ginger; it's also one of my favorites. This combination is a potassium powerhouse. For taste, you might add half a carrot and a green apple, or maybe a quarter of a lemon. If you don't do anything else to lose weight, at least drink one glass (8 to 10 ounces) of this juice every day and see the difference!

Overall Health Benefits

Eating enough fruits and vegetables can sometimes be difficult given the current demanding workloads and fast-paced lifestyles that we all live. Many of the people who have sat down with me ask me how I have enough time to meditate, juice, eat healthy, and work out. It's like I'm some kind of freak they found at a circus show. My response to them is simple.

A healthy lifestyle is the foundation for everything! The time I take to better my physical and mental health is the time that gives me my life-force for living an amazing life! The time I dedicate to my personal well-being gives me the unstoppable amounts of energy I have on a daily basis. It calms me, balances me, and the best part about it is that it keeps me super healthy. Without a healthy mind and body, we are unable to do all that is possible in this life. I get so much more accomplished in my day with this healthy foundation, and you will too, once you take the time to start.

What Should You Do First?

Lose the old mentality of eating animal protein, dairy, and pasta at every meal. Eating a sensible diet loaded in fruits and vegetables is a much healthier option. When you begin juicing, it does so much more for you than you could ever imagine.

Eating an abundance of uncooked live foods flushes your body of all the unwanted toxic chemicals that are in your body. It leaves you feeling refreshed, rejuvenated, and with a much greater sense of peace and well-being. If you have ever done yoga or gotten a back massage, the rejuvenated feeling you have after is similar to the effects of consuming a cup of juice.

The pure foods give your skin a healthy glow. Radiant, some say. The pure, live food also makes you smell cleaner, leaving you with naturally fresh breath. Sickly people with low immune systems usually report back to me with greater immune function and are in better shape after making juicing a regular part of their life. Getting sick is a thing of the past. One of the great things that I've found while juicing is that my mind is now in control of my body, and feeds it only what is necessary for the life of the trillions of cells in my body.

Sometimes, if my joints are sore from lifting, I'll have a certain juice (that can be found in this book) and my pains will go away. If my nose is plugged up from allergies and sinus pressure, I am now the holder of a secret juice recipe that will knock that symptom's socks off, getting my sinuses back in working order. If I feel like I'm coming down with a cold there are several juices that will give me all the immunity I need to push it out, making the illness powerless.

There is so much more your juice can do for you. Research points to certain types of vitamins and minerals in vegetables to be a great preventative measure for many deadly diseases. I'm therefore convinced that fresh vegetable juice is the answer to many of America's health problems. If you're overweight, juice. If you're tired, juice. Lost your shine, juice. You get my point.

The only thing you need to get started is a juicer.

Fruit Juice AND Veggie Juice

The recipes are the "juice" of this book. They are all meant to be mixed and matched. The way I like my juice may be completely different than the way you might like your juice. Plus, I've been juicing for a while now, so I'll double up on a lot of the recipes. My advice for you is to experiment with what you like.

There are some fundamental base mixtures that you can add to any veggie juice. There are also some things with which you want to proceed with caution (which are discussed later). Also, just because you are missing one ingredient doesn't mean you should run to the store or not drink the juice with whatever ingredients you have on hand. Juice it up anyway; you might surprise yourself.

Green Juices

Green juices are my go-to; my body just loves green drinks. You want to be careful in the beginning though. If you are not used to the greens, you could experience some gastric pain. Try mixing your green drinks with apple, cucumber, celery, or carrots at first.

You can juice (almost) anything green. Cucumbers and celery naturally give more juice than a lot of the leafy or coniferous vegetables—like broccoli, for example. It's always a good idea to make three-quarters of the cup a watery base by using cucumber or celery, and then the rest could be spinach, collard greens, cabbage, or beets. This will be the easier for your digestion at first. Eventually your body will

17

become used to the veggies and you will be able to drink an entire glass of spinach juice with no problems.

Fruit and Veggies Don't Always Mix

With a few exceptions like apples, lemons, and the occasional orange, it's best not to mix your fruits and veggies too much. The fruit will ferment and become much more difficult to break down. For example, what would normally take 30 minutes to process in your body will take up to three hours to process. It's even worse when you have fruit along with meat. This expands digestion time from three hours to eight, which is not good on anybody's system.

Fruit Juices – Recipe Time

1) Kick a Virus

An apple a day keeps the doctor away. There is truth to this in that the nutrients found in apples have been known to boost immune function. This is one of my favorite juices to have in the morning, and it will keep you from getting ill.

- 2 apples

- 1 orange

Peel the orange and cut the seeds out of the apple; they are not good for you. If the apples are not organic, don't even bother; they are loaded with chemicals. Get organic; it will cost you a little more, but the benefits are entirely worth it.

2) The Arouser

Skip the pills for erectile dysfunction and start juicing this. You will notice a *BIG* difference. Try adding a little apple juice for more of a complex taste.

- 2 bunches of black grapes

- 1-inch piece of ginger

- 4 strawberries (hulled)

- 1/2 cup of pitted black cherries

Many of the fruits and vegetables in these recipes will assist you in the bedroom because they enhance your circulatory system. If the blood is pumping, your sexual organs should be working as well. Some fruits and vegetables assist more than others, and this happens to be a combination that tastes great—and works great too!

3) Aches, Pains, and Sinus Drains
Simple Pineapple Juice

Simple, but amazing. Pineapple juice will cure aches and pains in your body. Sometimes I'll come back from the gym and rock out some APSD juice. If it's not organic, get rid of the skin. Cut the pineapple into long strips and juice it up. Make sure you wash the outside of the pineapple before you begin. Sometimes, when cutting, you can drag the nasty toxins inside to the meat of the pineapple.

4) Cantaloupe Juice
Cantaloupe supplies the body with beta-carotene and aids in digestion. Beta-carotene is the only source of carotene that can be turned into Vitamin A by the body. Vitamin A is absolutely critical to your health, assisting in your eyesight, bone growth, cell reproduction, and cell division. Vitamin A also helps maintain healthy skin and mucus membranes that defend against bacteria and viruses, and helps regulate the immune system.

- 1/4 of a cantaloupe

Cut the skin off and make the pieces small enough to pop in the juicer. Make sure when cutting the melon that you wash the skin first; again, you don't want to drag the nasties inside to the melon.

5) The Einstein

Grapefruit juice is great for controlling insulin levels on cheat days. It will give you energy as well as massive amounts of focus. This is a great pre-workout drink in the morning. I personally love grapefruit; it's my favorite fruit. It's low in carbs and calories, and can speed up your metabolism.

- 1 grapefruit

If organic, you can juice the skin. If not cut it off.

6) Pimp Juice

Feel like impressing your lady friend on a warm summer evening?

- 4 apricots
- 1 bunch of red grapes, preferably organic with stems
- 1 pear

Take the pits out of the apricots and cut the pear in half. Throw it in the juicer and turn on the music. It's about to go down.

7) R.E.L.A.X.

This juice always seems to bring me peace after a long day at work. It's also great for hydration, aches, and pains.

- Two 1-inch pineapple rounds, preferably organic
- 2 stalks of celery

If not organic, skin the pineapple.

8) Cantaloupe Apple

This supplies the body with a lot of beta-carotene, which is a disease-fighting substance. It also aids in digestion. The apple adds a great flavor along with additional health benefits

- A quarter of a full-sized melon
- 1 apple

9) Immunity Plus (Plus)

This drink will raise your immune system faster than you can say "I have immunity." Cranberries are great for your GI tract and for ridding your body of unwanted bacteria.

- 3 apples
- 1 cup cranberries

Cut the seeds out of the apple. (Organic apples only.) Put the rest of the fruit in the juicer.

10) Holistic Holiday Ginger Blast

This is a great juice to make for your guests and visitors around the holidays. Want to make sure your kids come home to visit you every year? Apples have a lot of great natural sugar and they aid in digestion. Make this juice and seal the deal.

- 3 apples
- 2 bunches of grapes
- 1 tiny piece of ginger
- 1 lemon

Peel the lemon and apples if they are not organic and get rid of the grape stems if not organic. Wash well.

11) Laugh Attack Juice

I was sitting at the kitchen table with a dear friend and this juice forced us to go into a fit of laughter for no reason. Try it and LYAO.

- 1 cup cranberries
- 1 bunch of green grapes, preferably organic, with stems
- One 1-inch pineapple round

If the grapes are not organic, remove the stems. If the pineapple is not organic, same deal; remove the rind.

Laughing can burn calories! It increases your T-cells and globulins, which aid your immune system. It also decreases

your stress hormones (cortisol, adrenaline, and dopac).
When we laugh, our body responds positively.

12) Brain Juice

I don't know what it is about this juice, but when I drink it
I feel like my mental acuity spikes instantly. It's probably the
B6 in the broccoli that gets my mind revved up.

- 1 broccoli shoot and floret diced up

- 1 cucumber

- 1 lemon

- 1/2 of a carrot

Dice the broccoli up so that it fits in the juicer. Peel the
lemon if it is not organic.

13) Attack The Day

Nothing gives me more energy in the morning than some
freshly squeezed high-quality orange juice. If you bought
your juicer only for oranges, you made a wise decision. Once
you try this you will NEVER want store-bought OJ again!

- 3 oranges

If they are not organic, make sure you peel them. If they
are organic, just throw them in the juicer. Eating a whole
orange can provide you with an abundance of fiber.
Sometimes I eat the orange as I would an apple.

One orange has over 170 phytonutrients and more than 60
flavonoids, many of which have been shown to have anti-

inflammatory, anti-tumor, and blood clot–inhibiting properties, as well as strong antioxidant effects.

14) Spartacus Juice

This is a great juice to drink before going into battle—or going to the gym. Whichever. With all of the vitamins of the orange and the insulin controls of the grapefruit, you can't go wrong drinking this pre-workout. It gives me loads of energy for battling against the evil bench press descending from Capua.

- 1 orange

- 1/4 grapefruit

- 1 lemon

If all your fruit is organic, leave the skin. If not, cut it off and process in the juicer.

15) Love Juice

If love had a flavor, this would be it. This has an unimaginable contrast between the apple, mango, and the pear. It's great for a dessert juice or in the morning after a little sleep-in time. You owe it to yourself to try it.

- 2 apples

- 1 pear

- 1/4 of a mango

- 3 strawberries

Drink it slowly and offer gratitude for the day. Peel the mango, and anything else that is not organic. Juice the mango first and the strawberries last to turn this into a tasty sunrise of love and adoration for the day.

16) Purple Passion Juice

This one is fun to make because of the pomegranate. It's perfect for a warm summer day. Put it on ice and give a glass to your neighbor. Who knows, maybe they will start mowing your lawn for you.

- 1/2 cup of pomegranate

- 1 apple

- 1 bunch of purple grapes (take the stems off if not organic)

Dice the pomegranate into pieces. If the juice is a little too bitter, take the seeds out.

Pomegranate juice is a rich source of sodium, and also contains a good amount of riboflavin, thiamine, niacin, Vitamin C, calcium, and phosphorous—a very powerful antioxidant.

17) Fruit Cocktail

This is a great-tasting juice that is great for cookouts and family get-togethers. If it's a hot summer day, you could always throw the fruit in a blender with some ice. Amazing!

- 1 orange

- 1/2 lime with skin

- 1/4 cup of blueberries

- 1 cup of sparkling mineral water

Peel the orange to rid the drink of the bitterness, and cut the lime in half so the juicer can handle it. If it is not organic, peel it. Pour the juice and add the sparkling water. Add lime or orange to garnish it.

18) Real Gatorade

This is a great drink to quench thirst during a long workout or run. Water is always the best, but most fruit is up to 60% water.

- 1 orange

- 1 lime

- 1 cup of water

This drink will hydrate you and give you some much-needed Vitamin C to ward off colds and keep you healthy. Put this on ice if it is hot outside.

I was talking to one of the vendors at a local farmers market and they told me it is best to eat the fruits that are in-season if you are trying to stay hydrated. The fruit in-season will have less packaging time and will offer the best hydrating benefits. Makes sense.

19) Miss Georgia Juice

Everyone loves a great-tasting supple peach. This drink tastes amazing! Peaches are a great source in Vitamin A, magnesium, and potassium. Grab yourself a glass of this and smile.

- 1 orange
- 1 peach
- 1/4 cup of mineral water
- 1 slice of orange to make it look cool

Pit the peach. Add the orange. Once you have your juice, add the mineral water and smile. I don't know why but this drink makes me smile, probably because it's also good for your teeth.

20) Ginger Ginger Ginger (or Ginger³)

Let me introduce you to my good friend Ginger. You have to start slow with her or she will bite you. She is great for pressing out toxins from your body and adding a little flair.

- 2 apples
- 1 orange
- 1 knob of ginger

Start this juice out with the apple and end with the apple. This will press the rest of the ginger out of the juicer. Peel the orange and apple if they are not organic.

21) Grapple Punch
This juice has a little punch to it that you will love.

- 1 bunch of green grapes

- 1 pineapple rind

- 1 lemon with skin if organic

- 1 cup mineral water

This is a great juice for you and the whole family. Remove the skin from the pineapple and the lemon if they are not organic. Put mineral water in. Why mineral water? Most water has to be processed, and during this processing it loses minerals. Mineral water, conversely, is usually found in a mineral-rich water source and has many health benefits.

22) Mountain "Drew"
This won't make you crash like the other green stuff. Sweet and sour, it's like drinking candy.

- 12 ounces of honeydew melon (Approximately a quarter of the melon)

- 1/2 of the lime with skin

Cut the honeydew into strips. Slice up the lime. Process the fruit all together.

23) California Love

Nothing can describe the flavor of California better than the lusciously passionate pineapple and the sexy succulent strawberries. Put these two together and you have California in a cup. Don't believe me? Try it. I dare you.

- 1 pineapple round

- 8 to 10 strawberries

If the pineapple is not organic, remove the skin. Process the fruit in the juicer. Enjoy the taste of California. If you don't live in California and would like to, imagine yourself on the beach while sipping on this cup of California heaven in hand.

24) Kiwi Kick Myself Silly

This one is like a karate convention in your mouth. The flavors jump-kick you in the tongue as you slurp down this bad boy.

- 1 bunch of green grapes

- 3 kiwis

- 1 orange

- 3 strawberries

Mmmmm. What more can I say? Make sure you peel your fruit if it is not organic (excluding the strawberries).

Laugh Fact: Laughter triggers the release of endorphins, the body's natural feel-good chemicals. Endorphins promote an overall sense of well-being and can even temporarily relieve pain.

25) Slap Happy Sammy

This drink will make you happy beyond measure. There is something about a mango that brings a sense of well-being into your life. Imagine for a moment the taste of the mango. Smiling yet?

- 1 mango
- 3 strawberries
- 1/2 lemon with skin
- 1 apple

Remove the skin from the mango, peel it in half, and remove the pit. Remove the skin on the apple if it is not organic. When you drink this, think back to a memory or a time where you felt really good about your life. Maybe there was a certain someone or something. Remember it.

26) Tenacious Titillating Tampa Juice

When I first moved from Michigan to Florida, I thought I died and went to heaven. Nothing against Michigan, it's a great place. It just didn't have fields upon fields of tropical fruit, unlike Tampa.

- 2 oranges
- 1/4 of a pineapple sliced long ways

Make sure to peel the orange and the pineapple, if they are not organic. Cut the orange so it can fit in your juicer.

27) Sweet and Sour Patch Morning

Mmmm. Enjoy the sweet flavor of the pineapple and the sour of the grapefruit.

- 1 pineapple round

- 1 grapefruit

This drink will help kick-start your day and give you massive amounts of energy for a morning workout. Try it and let me know how it works.

28) Zen Zinger

This is the juice of peace and tranquility. If you are experiencing any problems in your relationships, drink this juice and know that it will work out how it's supposed to.

- 2 golden delicious sweet apples

- 1 piece of ginger

- 3 kiwis

Garnish with a piece of sage, if you must.

Peel the fruit if any of it isn't organic. Start with an apple and end with an apple. When you drink this juice really center on that person who brings you a great deal of love in your life. Shift your awareness to someone who you are having trouble with and see that same type of love in that other person. Blanket them with love.

29) Fist Pumpin' Party Time!

Turn the music up and start dancing! This juice is guaranteed to put a little toot in your booty. (I don't really know what that means, but run with it anyway.)

- 1 pineapple round
- 1 orange
- 1/2 of a lemon, with skin

If the pineapple is not organic, remove and discard the skin. Same goes for the orange and lemon, or wash it really well.

30) Passion Juice

Whether you want to impress your significant other, or just love yourself, try this juice on for size. It will make your taste buds stand up and start hugging each other like crazed hippies.

- 1 pineapple round
- 1 bunch of grapes
- 8 strawberries (hulled)
- 1/2 of a lemon

Garnish with a piece of the strawberry

Peel the pineapple if it is not organic. Remove the stems from the grapes and cut the lemon in half.

31) Papple Juice

This is a combination of two of my favorite fruits—apple and pear. Mmmm. This is a great juice to drink while eating with cheese.

- 2 apples

- 1 pear

Peel both if they are not organic and cut the seeds out of the apple. Enjoy this over ice on a warm summer day.

32) Pink Panther Flush

This is another sweet and sour classic of mine. Great before the gym or if you just want a little hop in your step. This juice will help control your insulin levels while getting your sugar from the apples and using the ginger to press out toxins. Classic!

- 2 apples

- 1/2 grapefruit

- 1 ginger

Make sure you peel the apples if they are not organic. Put an apple in first and last.

33) San Francisco Fog Basher

Great drink in the morning to get your heart pumping and your mind awake. If you are experiencing lack of focus, this is a great drink. The lemon will help alkalize your body as well.

- 2 apples
- 8 strawberries
- 1 lemon

Peel the apples if they are not organic. Cut the seeds out from the apple core as well. Wash your lemon with some veggie wash or soak it in grapefruit juice and water.

34) Drew Juice

This is my favorite fruit juice. First of all, I love the flavor of apple juice, and when the ginger is added it gives it an amazing kick. Of course, I'm the guy who would chew on ginger if it were laying around. This is a great one for cold prevention, as well.

- 4 apples
- 1 ginger piece

Try this juice out and you will know what I'm talking about. Make sure you peel your apple if it is not organic, and get rid of the seeds in the core.

35) Lucy Juice

I have a friend and this is her absolute all-time favorite. It's a simple mix and can be mixed with champagne. (That's the way she likes it.)

- 1 bunch of purple grapes

- 8 strawberries

Get rid of the stems if the grapes are not organic. Pour a little champagne on top to turn this into a party drink or if you need a little hair-o'-the-dog.

36) Sunrise Juice

There's nothing more magnificent or captivating than waking up every morning to catch a good sunrise. I've been in this discipline for years, and many times I like to have this type of juice accompany me.

- 2 apples

- 4 strawberries

- 1 lemon

- 1 handful of cherries (from Michigan if you can)

Cut the skin off the apple if it is not organic and wash the rest of your fruit. If you are fortunate enough to have a good view of the sun in the morning, drink this to salute it and give thanks to the sun for providing you with light and warmth throughout the day.

37) Watermelon Kidney Flush

This is a great juice to detoxify your kidneys and leave you feeling refreshed and rejuvenated. Very sugar-based, so you might want to do one part water to one part juice.

- 1/2 of a baby watermelon

Dice up the watermelon to fit in the juicer. Make sure you wash the skin well. This is where the majority of the nutrients are held.

38) Lemmy the Apple

- 2 apples
- 1 lemon
- 1-inch slice of ginger

If the apples are organic, juice them with their skins on. The skin is the most abundant area of the apple for flavonoid content. This will produce cloudy but more nutritious (and still delicious) apple juicer recipes. This healthy juicer recipe also makes a great remedy for colds. Peel the lemon if it is not organic.

39) Berry Medley

- 2 cups of strawberries
- 2 cups of blueberries
- 1-1/2 cups of raspberries

Berries are among the quickest and easiest of fruits to juice. The only prepping they need is a quick rinse.

Strawberries are a small exception, as they will need to be topped before juicing.

40) Breakfast Bounce

This will put a little bounce in your step.

- 3 oranges

- 1 grapefruit

Make sure you peel the oranges and the grapefruit. Place fruit in the juicer and enjoy.

41) Kiwi Blue

This is a classic for anyone who loves a sweet little treat.

- 3 kiwis

- 2 cups of blueberries

Peel kiwis and wash berries, juice, enjoy.

Blue fruits, such as the highly esteemed blueberries, contain a wide variety of phytochemicals. Anthocyanins give blueberries their amazing color. Blueberries contain other phytochemicals that can improve memory. They are also a great anti-aging fruit.

42) Fresh Lemonade

If this were sold on the street corner by the neighbor's kid, it would be worth more than a quarter. You really can't beat this recipe.

- 2 or 3 large lemons
- 1/2 cup of water

(Optional: Add an apple to sweeten, instead of sugar)

Peel lemons and cut stem of apple. (Swap out 1 lemon for 1 lime and bingo, you've got limeade). Add ice on those hot days.

43) The Silent Strawberry

Love this combination! The strawberry is subtle and it just sneaks up on you.

- 1/3 cup of strawberries
- 1 cup of blueberries
- 2 apples

Wash all the ingredients well and juice.

Red fruits such as strawberries contain the phytochemical lycopene that gives them their red color. Lycopene has been shown to help prevent prostate cancer and heart disease.

44) Pear and Kiwi Juice

This is a great energy juice and is high in Vitamin C.

- 2 kiwis

- 2 pears

Peel kiwis and remove pear stems. People will really enjoy this juice.

45) Melon Medley

Like melons on a hot summer day, you will enjoy this even more. Tantalize your taste buds with this juice. Don't say I didn't warn you.

- 1/2 of a watermelon

- 1/2 of a honeydew melon

- 1/2 of a cantaloupe

Remove rinds and seeds (except for watermelon seeds). Put contents in the juicer and enjoy.

46) Tropical Fruit Juice Recipes

My mother loves this one. She is up in Michigan most of the year but when she visits me in Florida I serve this juice.

- 1 orange

- 1 kiwi

- 1/2 mango

- Sparkling mineral water

Peel all the fruits, and also pit the mango. Pour the juice in a large glass, fill to the top with sparkling water, and serve.

47) Kidney Cleanse

This juice has been proven to clean your kidneys out. Careful on the watermelon; it is really sweet.

- 2 apples

- 3 1/2 watermelon pieces with rind (About an inch a piece)

Wash your fruit. Even slicing a melon that is nonorganic can pull the toxins from the outside in. Cut the apples into narrow wedges and juice with the watermelon pieces. Juice, and enjoy healthy kidneys.

48) The Pain Reducer

This juice will help relieve you from aches and pains.

- 1 lemon

- 1 orange

- 2 hard pears

- 2 apples

Peel orange and lemon, remove pear and apple stems, and juice.

49) S² (Supreme Splendid)

Once this juice hits your lips the word "splendid" will come out of your mouth. Promise.

- 1 orange, peeled and sectioned

- 1 cup fresh pineapple, cubed, skin removed

- 5 strawberries

Peel orange and pineapple, and top the strawberries. Process the fruit in a juicer and serve. You are going to love this juice.

50) Five-star Tropical Lineup

Nothing says the tropics like this juice. The combination of guava and mango is amazing. Remember, I'm not neglecting anything from the rest of this all-star cast. You are going to become addicted to this juice.

- 1 mango

- 1 large orange

- 1 pineapple slice

- 1 papaya

- 1 guava

Peel and remove all pits and seeds. This is another favorite juicer recipe of mine. Awesome on a hot day with ice!

Vegetable Juice Recipes

This is where the start of lifelong health and anti-aging begins. I hope you are as excited as I am. Fruit juices are great for overall health and well-being, but nothing says, "I'm going to live to be 200!" like a good green drink.

Vegetables are the building blocks to life. They supply your body with all of the necessary vitamins and minerals. Did you know that there is actually more protein in most leafy greens—like spinach and collard greens—than there is in a steak? These greens are 45% protein. However, you have to eat a lot of spinach to get the same amount that is in that piece of animal flesh. Why not juice it instead? Plus, the juice actually tastes better!

Some of these recipes will require a little bit of fruit for taste, although it's not necessary. These are my recipes after many wins, and an occasional loss here or there. I remember a few juices that no one would drink!

Most of these juices will be absolutely delicious, and if by chance you don't like a recipe and want to alter it, feel free. This book is to help get you started and give you ideas.

1) Recharge Your Alkaline Battery

Do you have gas in your pants? Feel tired or acidic? Maybe you've had one too many coffees today? This juice will help you bounce back quickly.

- handful of red cabbage

- 1 cucumber

- handful of spinach

- 1 lemon

Cut the skin off the cucumber if it is not organic; it's good to get rid of the wax they put on it. If you have the option, buy plastic-wrapped, pesticide-free cucumbers. Juice the rest of the veggies as normal.

2) Anti-Ulcer / Probiotic Juice

Looking to balance your system out? This juice will do it. When the going gets tough, the tough get juicing. There are all kinds of probiotics in this glass of greens. Great drink for clearing free radicals and disease prevention.

- 1/4 red cabbage

- 2 handfuls of spinach

- 4 collard green leaves

- 4 stalks of celery

Wash all of your veggies and start juicing.

Probiotics are live microorganisms that, when administered in adequate amounts, confer a health benefit on the host. I like to think of probiotics as little bodyguards in my intestinal track. If something nasty comes in, they clean up the mess.

3) Anti-Acne—Miracle Skin

This juice has been used to clear the skin from within. It is great for anyone who spends hundreds of dollars per year on late-night infomercial pimple creams.

- 6 carrots
- 1/2 green bell pepper

Cut the tops off the carrots and bell pepper, rinse, and drink. When drinking this juice, visualize the nutrients furnishing enough nutrients and energy to rid your body of the toxins causing these blemishes. See them going away.

4) Life Regenerator Blood Boost

Drink this juice to purify and give your blood the iron it needs. A 180-gram serving of boiled spinach contains 6.43 milligrams of iron, whereas one 170-gram ground hamburger patty contains at most 4.42 milligrams.

- 5 carrots
- 1 handful of parsley
- 2 radishes
- 6 spinach leaves
- 4 lettuce leaves
- 1 piece of ginger

Trim the tops of the carrots off and wash all your vegetables. Put them in the juicer and enjoy. Drink this juice slowly. I usually spend 15 minutes drinking a juice like this. You've heard the saying, "chew your juice."

Ever wonder why Popeye was so strong? Iron is the main ingredient in hemoglobin, which is found in red blood cells and is responsible for carrying oxygen throughout the body. Without enough iron, the body is unable to produce enough hemoglobin and, as a result, muscles get less oxygen, which reduces the body's energy.

5) Body Purifier

I drink this juice to flush out the necessary toxins and give my heart a boost.

- 2 carrots

- 1 cucumber

- 1/2 cauliflower

- 1/2 of a beet

Cut the top off the carrots and peel the skin off of the cucumber if it is not organic. Many times, if the beet is not organic, the chemicals will be at the base where the beet and the stems connect. Make sure it is clean or cut it off completely.

6) Bone Builder

Strong bones are quintessential to good health. Many vegetables take on the shape and form of what they are good for in the body. If you look at celery, it looks like your bones. So, as you might guess, celery is the chosen vegetable here.

- 8 stalks of celery

- 2 carrots

- 1 bunch of parsley

- 1 lemon

Dice the celery up small enough to fit in the blender, and trim the tops off the carrot. Peel them if they are not organic and wash your vegetables.

Diet/nutrition is the key ingredient to great heart health. Adding carrots and cauliflower are two good things you can do, being low in salt and easy to tolerate. Stick to a raw diet as much as possible. This will allow your heart to heal the quickest.

7) Capri Kiddie Juice

When kids won't eat their veggies, it's because they like sweet stuff. So this is your "healthy" key to sweeten up the green goodness of the broccoli and cucumber.

- 1 broccoli floret

- 1 cucumber

- 2 apples

Just be careful not to give them too much apple juice because they could start running around the house at an accelerated rate. Trim all of the vegetables so they fit in the juicer. Peel them if they are not organic.

8) Simply Green Machine

Green drinks are my favorite, and more often I go to this type of juice. Enjoy this one. The parsley is great for eliminating bad breath and body odor.

- 1 cup of spinach

- 2 cups of kale

- 2 cups of parsley

- 1 cucumber

- 3 celery stalks

Add a little garlic and/or ginger if you like. Wash thoroughly and juice.

Parsley is a good source of folic acid, one of the most important B vitamins. It plays a lot of key roles in your body, but chief among them is your cardiovascular health. The flavonoids in parsley have been shown to function as antioxidants that combine with highly reactive oxygen-containing molecules (called oxygen radicals) and help prevent oxygen-based damage to cells.

In addition, extracts from parsley have been used in animal studies to help increase the antioxidant capacity of the blood reducing tumors.

9) Cukeapple Zippy

This has a great zip to it. I love ginger in my juices.

- 2-1/2 apples
- 1/2 cucumber
- 1-inch piece of ginger

Remove apple stems and juice everything together.

10) Heaven Sent

You know anything with the word "heaven" in the title has to be amazing. Just try it and tell me what you think.

- 1 cup of spinach
- 1/2 cucumber
- 2 stalks of celery including leaves
- 3 carrots
- 1/2 apple

Wash everything thoroughly, top the carrots, remove apple stem, juice, and enjoy.

11) The Cucapple

Simple yet satisfying, hydrating and energy-packed.

- 1/2 cucumber
- 2 apples

Remove the stems from the apples, cut the cucumber in half, and juice. The nice thing about both apples and cucumbers is that you get a lot of juice out of them. This is great when you just need something quick.

12) Parsley Pump Up

This is one of my favorite juices as well. There is nothing like fresh parsley in a juice to clean out your system.

- 1 cup of parsley

- 1/2 apple

- 2 carrots

- 3 celery stalks

Wash all thoroughly, remove apple stem, top the carrots, juice, and enjoy!

13) Bless My Eyes, For Now I Can See!

Carrots and kale, what more can I say? Did Bugs Bunny ever wear glasses? No. Did he have X-ray vision like Superman? No. Will you have X-ray vision? Probably not.

- 6 carrots

- 1 cup of kale

That's right; carrots are great for your eyes! Okay, it's not the actual carrot; it is the beta-carotene that is *in* the carrot. When it is converted to Vitamin A in the liver, it is then transformed to rhodopsin, a purple-colored pigment that is used at night to see. Beta-carotene is a powerful antioxidant that aids against macular degeneration, which happens to be the leading cause of blindness in the elderly.

14) Liver Life

Clean your liver and everything else.

- 1/2 beet with greens

- 3 apples

Wash all thoroughly, remove apple stems, and put the half- beet in.

15) Green Juice Recipes Energizer

This one is a real blast, brimming with goodness. It's one of my favorite weight-loss juices as well.

- 2 apples

- 1/2 cucumber

- 1/2 lemon (peeled)

- 1/2 cup of kale

- 1/2 cup of spinach

- 1/4 bunch of celery

- 1/4 bulb of fennel

- 1-inch piece of ginger

- 1/4 head of romaine lettuce

Kale is high in beta-carotene. Kale also has a significant supply of vegetable protein that is amazing for your body. Next time you are at the market, look for kale's healthy but ignored cousins—Swiss chard, mustard greens, and collards.

16) My Memory, Oh My!

This juice will activate your brain to help recall memories from the past. This is great for students who are about to take an exam. The mint is the key.

- 1 cucumber

- 1 carrot

- 1 green apple

- 1/4 cup parsley

- 1/4 cup mint

- 1 stalk of celery

- 1/2-inch inch of fresh ginger

- 1/2 of a lemon (peeled)

Wash and peel all of your nonorganic vegetables. Cut up to fit in the juicer and enjoy.

17) Energizer Bunny

If you are in an energy slump, this is the juice for you. Get ready to turn your 9-volt back on. This juice will get you revved up and ready to face the day.

- 2 carrots

- 1 broccoli floret

- 2 handfuls of spinach

- 1/2 of a beet

- 1 lemon

You will love this juice. It's one of my personal favorites. Trim up the carrots so they fit in the juicer. If the lemon is not organic, trim the skin off that as well.

18) Sleep Better Sally

I sometimes drink this juice if I'm having trouble sleeping. It not only helps you sleep, it cleans your system out while you drift off into la-la land. Magnesium and zinc are vitamins that help you slumber. Both spinach and kale are high in magnesium and zinc.

- 2 handfuls of spinach
- 4 stalks of celery
- 3 kale leafs
- 1 lemon

Great natural detox, I make sure to brush my teeth after this drink and before bed because the lemon has acid in it that is bad for your teeth enamel, so you don't want it sitting on your teeth while sleeping.

19) C2L

This juice calms me and gives me focused energy throughout the night. If you've had a long day at the office, but still have a busy night ahead of you and need to get lots of stuff done, this is the juice for you.

- 1/4 red cabbage

- 2 carrots

- 1 lemon

Drink this juice slowly so your body absorbs the nutrients. Trim the tops off the carrots and dice them up to fit them in the juicer. I drink this after a long workout and it eliminates a lot of the fatigue I'm experiencing.

Cabbage is amazing! It has the ability to aid you in your digestion process. It is also rich in antioxidants and loaded with anti-inflammatory effects.

20) Apple and Cauliflower Juice

Normally I'm not fond of the way cauliflower tastes, but when you release a few magical golden delicious apples into the center of it, you will be very satisfied.

- 3 apples

- 1/2 cauliflower head

Peel the apple if it is not organic, and make sure you wash the cauliflower thoroughly.

21) Carrot and Celery Juice

Celery is a great base juice for any of your mixes. It doesn't hold a lot of flavor but it is amazing for your bones. When you add the carrot to the celery juice, it gives you the flavor you are looking for.

- 6 celery stalks

- 3 carrots

Trim up your veggies so they fit in the juicer; remember to cut the top off of the carrots and wash thoroughly.

22) The Orange and Green Mohawk

This brightly colored drink is amazing for your digestive tract, and it tastes great too!

- 4 carrots

- 1/2 beet

- 1 handful of parsley

Trim the tops off of the carrots and beet. Wash your veggies.

23) Cauliflower Broccoli Monster

This is a drink that will leave you feeling strong. There is no wonder in it either; there is a ton of phosphorus in both cauliflower and broccoli.

- 3 carrots

- 1/2 broccoli floret

- 1/2 cauliflower head

Trim the top off the carrot and dice your veggies up enough to fit in your juicer. Bookend your juice with the carrots to maximize your juice efforts. When drinking this juice, really feel the protein from the broccoli go into your cells.

24) The Ripley (Believe It or Not)

This is the juice that could have saved Mr. Ripley's life, and has been one of his all-time favorites since he started. It also helps that it doesn't cost an arm and a leg to make.

- 3 apples

- 3 carrots

Peel your apples if they are not organic, and remove the seeds. Trim the tops from the carrots and, "Voilà!"

25) Lake City Winter Bluice

This is a drink that will warm you up and get your blood boiling. It's especially great in my hometown, Lake City, Michigan. What better way to warm up your body functions than by heating them up with some nutritious, bold and tasty juice. This juice will chase away the winter blues.

- 2 carrots
- 1/2 beet
- 1 handful of parsley
- 1 handful of cilantro
- 1 pinch of cayenne pepper
- 1 tomato
- 1 cup tonic

Wash all of your vegetables thoroughly. Trim the tops off of the carrots and the beat. Put the parsley and cilantro in toward the middle. Once the juice is complete, add the tonic and you are off. Garnish with a pickle, if you must.

26) Cholesterol Cruncher

This juice will kick your cholesterol to the curb.

- 2 bok choy
- 8 asparagus
- 1 apple
- 1-inch piece ginger
- 2 handfuls of spinach

Wash all your veggies thoroughly. Dice your apple into pieces, remove the seeds, and peel it if it is not organic. When you drink this juice, imagine your blood cleaning out and getting healthier. This visualization technique will be helpful in the healing process.

27) Blood Infusion

This is a power-packed drink for your blood and heart. It opens up your circulatory system and both beetroot and greens are powerful cleansers and builders of the blood.

- 1/2 beet

- 2 leafs red chard

- 2 carrots

- 1/2 cucumber

- dash of cayenne

Wash the beets and trim the tops off, clean the red chard, and cut the tops off the carrots. Enjoy the sweet spice of this drink.

28) Carrot Spinach Juice (GI Tract Special)

This juice helps with digestion and is packed with vitamins. Powerful stuff! It goes well with your meal.

- 4 or 5 carrots

- 3 handfuls of spinach

- 1 broccoli floret

Trim the tops off of the carrots and wash the spinach.

29) Stomach Soother

Any juice containing cabbage soothes the stomach as long as it is mixed with a milder juice.

- 1/2 of a cabbage
- 4 carrots
- 2 apples
- 1 piece of ginger root

Trim the cabbage and carrots so that they can fit in the juicer. Remove the apple seeds.

30) White Eye Juice

Ever wonder why people who eat only raw food have white eyes? This is one of my secret juices that will clean your eyes. Normally when a person's eyes are red, it's due to stress or a stressed out liver. This will detox your liver and get it working for you again.

Start by avoiding alcohol, refined sugar, and trans fat. You want to clean your liver as much as possible.

- 2 leaves of collard greens
- 4 carrots
- 2 leaves of kale
- 2 mustard green leaves
- 1 lemon

Wash all your vegetables thoroughly. Trim the tops of the carrots. Peel the lemon if it is not organic.

The liver is the largest gland in the body. It eliminates toxic chemicals in your blood. It also aids in the absorption of your vitamins and minerals. Look at the liver like your body's internal filter, keeping the good and eliminating the bad. Detoxify by metabolizing and/or secreting drugs, alcohol, and environmental toxins.

31) House Salad Juice

This is a great juice to drink on a day when you want to feel lean. Maybe you are going to the beach tomorrow and want to look good in that new bikini.

- 3 carrots
- 1/2 head of lettuce
- 1/4 red cabbage

Wash all of your veggies. Trim the tops off the carrots. Dice up the lettuce and cabbage to fit in your juicer.

32) Got Gray Hair?

This juice will you keep the gray away to come out another day!

- 1/4 head of lettuce
- 1/4 head of cabbage
- 2 carrots

Wash all your veggies. Trim the cabbage and the lettuce to fit inside the juicer.

33) Super Green Machine

This juice will get you cut up. When you are done drinking this juice, you will look like you dunked your abs in a bucket of knives. Not really, but you get my point.

- 1 cucumber

- 2 handfuls of spinach

- 1 broccoli floret

- 2 leafs of kale

- 1 lemon

Trim the skin off of your cucumber if it is not organic. Dice up the rest of your veggies so they fit in the juicer. Peel the skin off of the lemon if it is not organic.

34) Hair Rejuvenator

Worried about losing your hair? Ever notice how alfalfa sprouts look surprisingly like hair follicles? There are all types of people out there promising to re-grow your hair, so why not try this organic, chemical-free one?

- 1 handful of alfalfa sprouts

- 4 lettuce leaves

- 1 lemon

- 1 cucumber

Trim the tops off your carrots, and wash all the lettuce leaves and sprouts. Put the sprouts inside the lettuce leaf and juice.

35) Muscle Cramp Stopper

When cramping starts to happen, potassium can help aid you in muscle rejuvenation.

- 2 carrots

- 6 asparagus

- 6 celery stalks

Trim the tops off the carrots and wash your vegetables.

36) Infection Fighting and Virus Beater

Garlic is a natural antibiotic; it will help ward off any unwanted colds. Be careful not to add too much garlic, especially if you are going out on a hot date.

- 1 garlic clove

- 2 apples

- 2 carrots

- 1/2 beet

- 1 lemon

Skin the garlic and trim the tops off the carrots. Cut off the top of the beets and peel the lemon.

37) Jicima Juice

Are you afraid to admit that you don't know what jicama (pronounced "hik-a-muh") is? Well, fear not, I had no clue either. But it is very refreshing in juice!

- 1 slice of jicama

- 3 carrots

- 1/2 beet

1 handful of parsley

Jicama is great for an upset stomach. Make sure you wash all your vegetables, and slice the tops off of your carrots.

38) Hopeful Heart

Great detoxifier juice and amazing for your heart and liver!

- 3 apples

- 1/2 beet

Wash all your vegetables. Peel the apple if it is not organic. Cut the top off of the beet and let the juicing begin.

39) L.A. Lung Juice

This is a great juice for detoxifying your lungs. If you are a little congested, this could free up some of the mucus that is clogging you up.

- 1 handful of parsley

- 4 celery stalks

- 4 sprigs of watercress

Wash your vegetables accordingly. Process them in the juicer.

Watercress—gram for gram—has a higher nutritional value then apples, broccoli, and tomatoes. The watercress has more C, B1, B6, K, E, iron, calcium, magnesium, manganese, and zinc. Only raw broccoli has more Vitamin C and magnesium.

Watercress is bursting with beta-carotene and Vitamin A—which, as well as being important antioxidants, are also needed for healthy skin and eyes—containing more than four times the amount of the other "power" foods. No wonder it is good for your lungs. Next time you are at the store pick up some watercress.

40) Bone and Nail Health

The calcium content in these vegetables will strengthen your bones and nails.

- 1/2 cucumber

- 2 kale leaves

- 1/2 green bell pepper

- 1 lemon

Wash and trim your vegetables. Make sure you peel the lemon and cucumber if they are not organic.

41) Stamina Boost

The magnesium in this juice will provide long-standing stamina. This juice adds intensity and extra "oomph!" to your workouts.

- 1/2 cucumber

- 2 bok choy

- 4 carrots

Trim the tops off the carrots and peel your cucumber if it is not organic.

42) Pancreases Pump

Pump up the pancreas with this juice. The pancreas is in charge of insulin production. Insulin is responsible for breaking down glucose in your body. Pump up your insulin and burn body fat effectively and efficiently. What is good for the pancreas is good for the entire body.

- 2 apple
- 4 carrots
- 2 lettuce leaves
- 4 string beans
- 2 Brussels sprouts
- 1 handful of sprouts

Make sure you wash all your vegetables. Put the sprouts inside the lettuce leaf and juice.

43) Go-Go Juice

This is a great juice to have in the morning before or after a workout. This is one of my favorite juices, getting me revved up and ready for the day. Simple to make but the rewards you get from the nutrients are incredible.

- 1/2 cucumber
- 1 lemon
- 1 ginger piece
- 2 apples
- 4 celery stalks

44) MEGA GREEN MAN (a.k.a. THE DAY SLAYER)

If you are in an energy slump, this is the juice for you, getting you revved up and ready to slay the day.

- 2 carrots
- 1 broccoli floret
- 2 collard green leaves
- 1 ginger knuckle
- 2 handfuls of spinach
- 1 handful of dandelion greens
- 1/4 beet
- 1 lemon

This juice is one of my personal favorites. Trim up the carrots so they fit in the juicer. If the lemon is not organic, trim the skin off that as well. Wash the rest of the vegetables with "veggie wash" and get ready to dominate life.

45) Hot Stuff

Jalapeno is great for opening up your circulatory system ridding it from toxins.

- 1 jalapeno
- 1 cucumber
- 1/2 red bell pepper
- 1/2 beet

Wash your vegetables, and peel the cucumber if it is not organic. Place the vegetables in the juicer.

46) Red Devil

Like spicy food? This juice is for you. Imagine your favorite Mexican dish in a glass. This one is great for headaches and congestion. I also love this one due to the fast-acting metabolism boost in the jalapeno and cayenne.

- 1 jalapeno

- 1 beet

- 2 leaves Swiss red chard

- 1 lemon

- 1 dash of cayenne

Wash your vegetables. Cut the top off of the beet. Juice your vegetables and put a little cayenne pepper when stirring this juice up. (Stir up the juice with the pepper when done.)

Spicy foods can kick the metabolism into high gear. Juicing a tablespoon of chopped red or green chili pepper can temporarily boost your metabolic rate by 23 percent. This lasts for 30 to 45 minutes after eating.

Capsaicin (the chemical that puts the spice in your life and melts away body fat) also helps to inhibit inflammation and is beneficial in the treatment of arthritis and nerve disorders.

47) Hellatios Habanero

This one is at a Level 10 on the hot gauge. If you like a burning sensation in your mouth, then this one is it. Habanero peppers contain amino acids that help regulate body functions. They contain Vitamin A and C.

- 1 lemon

- 1 habanera

- 1/2 cucumber

- 4 carrots

- 1 handful of parsley

Granted it's a little spicy, but it's an amazing juice to clean out your liver. Peel the lemon and trim the tops off of the carrots. Enjoy.

48) Sexy Skin Sap

This juice is great for colds and nausea. It is also great for smoother, age-defying skin.

- 1 lemon

- 1/2 cucumber

- 1 bunch of watercress

- 2 carrots

- 1 ginger root

Wash all your vegetables and peel the cucumber and lemon if they are not organic.

49) Skin Revival

Are you ready to help diminish those fine lines and wrinkles? Have you been spending countless dollars on high-end beauty products and facials? Well get ready to feast your face on this.

- 2 leaves of chard

- 1 lemon

- 2 carrots

- 1/2 green bell pepper

- 2 leaves of kale

Wash your vegetables. Cut the tops off of the carrots and peel the lemon if it is not organic. Process in the juicer.

50) Beet the Street Juice

This is a juice I like to drink before a long run. This gives me sustainable energy and it tastes delicious. Be careful at first, though, if you are not used to beets.

- 1 beet

- 4 celery stalks

- 1 lemon

Cut the tops off of the lemon and beet. Peel the lemon if it is not organic and process your vegetables in the juicer.

51) Zip Zap Zing Juice

This a powerful juice to drink before a meeting and when you need extra brainpower. This will give your brain the zip-zing that it needs to focus on the task at hand and get stuff done.

- 1/2 cucumber

- 1/2 beet

- 2 stalks of celery

- 1/2 lemon

- 1 ginger root

- 1 handful cilantro

- 1 handful of chard

Wash your vegetables. Place the herbs in the juicer halfway through to get the maximum benefit of the nutrients. Peel the lemon and cucumber if they are not organic. Cut the tops off of the cucumber and the beet. Process in the juicer.

52) Nite Nite Sleep Tight Juice

Having trouble sleeping? This will have you falling to sleep faster than you can count five sheep.

- 2 bok choy

- 1 cucumber

- 2 handfuls of spinach

- 1 lemon

Wash your vegetables. Peel the cucumber and lemon if they are not organic. Put the rest of the vegetables in the juicer and say good night. Z-z-z-z-z . . .

53) The Situation Six-Pack

Get ready to pop out that sexy six-pack when chugging this alkaline goody.

- 2 carrots
- 1 cucumber
- 1/2 beet with greens
- 3 handfuls of spinach
- 1/2 lemon

Cut the tops off the carrots and peel the cucumber and lemon if they are not organic.

54) Extreme Juice

This juice is extreme! Coming out of the gates, we have the jalapeño that will open up your circulatory system and get you ready for the day—or anything else!

- 1 jalapeño
- 1 cucumber
- 2 handfuls of spinach
- 1 lemon
- 3 mustard leaves

Make sure to peel the lemon if it is not organic, and the cucumber. This should make an 8-ounce glass of juice.

One natural ingredient in green juice recipes is chlorophyll, which is the product of plants turning light into energy for insects and animals to eat. Without chlorophyll, life as we know it would not exist. It has powerful detoxifying principles. It's great for the liver, which is necessary in purifying your body. Chlorophyll can also improve our blood quality due to its molecular makeup, similar to hemoglobin. It helps increase red blood cell count and increases the movement of oxygen throughout our blood. It also helps the repair and growth of all tissues in the body.

Parting Thoughts
You Make the Difference

"It was your character that got you out of bed,
commitment that moved you into action, and
ongoing discipline that enabled you to follow
through and reach your destiny."

—Drew Canole

When I first started my exercise transformation, my body fat was a solid 17 percent. My exercise transformation started with going to the gym twice daily, where I pushed my body to the limits and maintained a healthy diet. It all resulted in trimming my stomach to a lean 12% in 90 days. However, when I started juicing daily, my gains increased substantially, continually lowering my body fat while building lean muscle.

Once the juice transformed my body's reception of nutrients, it enabled me to press out the water and toxins that were holding me back from my ultimate goal. This eventually allowed me to realize my potential sustainability of a body fat at or below 7 percent.

Maybe having a low body fat percentage is not your ideal goal, but optimum health is. If this is the case, the juice will help. However, exercise is a must! Even if it's just walking at first, you must take action. The hardest part for most people in the beginning of a regimen is to build up sustainability in doing so. The following five actions have helped me tremendously with my discipline and in my ability to take action.

Stop being a victim

Everyone who has a problem with their weight, overall physical health, or physique, more often than not blames it on something outside of themself. "I'm this way because of this."

Do you often find yourself saying, or thinking these insignificant thoughts?

It's a hard pill to swallow when you realize *you're* the creator of everything that comes into your experience. Once you take ownership of it, you will begin to free yourself from all of the restrictions you've come up with in the past.

By not taking ownership, you end up rationalizing everything by telling yourself it isn't your fault and there isn't anything you can do about it, which ends up stunting your potential. For example, those extra three cookies you had Sunday after dinner. You might rationalize this indulgence by saying, "It's okay, I'll just do more cardio in the morning." The morning comes and the cardio never happens; sleep was too important, you have an extra long day at work, etc.

You must take ownership and responsibility of the time you have in the present moment. Stop procrastinating. Once you master this discipline, you can get outside of your physical body and move this discipline to higher realms. Until then, you will be stuck on the island of blame with no escape.

Don't let yourself be a victim. Far too many people have the victim mentality. Don't try to rationalize why you are where you are right now by blaming other people and ill circumstances. Admit to yourself that you are in the situation you are in it because of what YOU'VE done and no one else. Take control of your life. You can't go back to the past, but today you can start to create a new, healthy, enduring, and vigorous life.

Put Your Workouts on Automation

Wouldn't it be great to have your Avatar venture into the gym every morning for you? For me personally, I have a morning routine that I follow. Perhaps this will encourage you to do the same.

5:30: Wake up! (Ten minutes of gratitude. Drink 1 liter of water and grapefruit juice, equal parts. All of my gym clothes are laid out ready to go. The easier I make it, the less I will fail.)

6:00: Gym time. I have a timer set to give me 1 hour in the gym.

7:00–7:15: Back home; juice time with a giant green drink.

7:30: Meditate and read for 1 hour.

8:30: Netti Pot, steam, and shower.

9:00: Time to play. This is when I get to go to work.

The point of the automated morning routine is to form a lifelong habit of doing this. I call it a success ritual. When I miss a day or when I'm traveling, I miss my ritual because it sets me up for success every day. It wasn't always this way, I must admit. There was a time in my life when I DID NOT look forward to going to the gym, or even getting out of bed for that matter.

Set a Goal

If you really want to take your game to the next level, create urgency in your situation. Set a goal to run a race or some other type of competition. Far too often, we have no goals or plan, and we fail. Winston Churchill said it best: "By failing to prepare, you are preparing to fail." Create a plan and stick with it. Write out what you would like to accomplish—even if it is walking to the mailbox in two weeks, write it out.

Change Your Environment

It has been said that if you hang out with wolves you will become one. Or if you lie with dogs, you will get fleas. In any type of new regime, some of the people in your life could subconsciously be holding you back. Understand that this behavior is not them; it is their own ego that is doing this. I'll make a bold claim: I can tell a person's fitness level by seeing five of the people they hang out with in their lives the most.

Who are you spending your time with?

Every cell in your body craves homeostasis, or balance. When you start to do something that is outside of the norm, some of the people in your life may not approve. Let's face it, not many of my friends crave broccoli and carrot juice at 6 a.m. before a workout on a Saturday morning.

What do you do when faced with this situation?

This is the best part—you make new friends. You don't have to get rid of your current friends; you just supplement them with these new individuals. In doing so, make sure they are the type of people who love broccoli and carrot juice, or at least accept you for you.

Turn it into a game (advanced tactic).

One of my favorite things to do is to turn my routine into a game. I have a Gym Boss interval timer that I use to monitor my time. This puts me in a mode of "watching the stop clock." It's similar to the way a basketball player watches the clock at the end of each quarter and through the game, increasing his chances to win. The timer sits next to my bed and as soon as my gratitude moment is over, I jump out of bed excited and ready to take on the day.

Throughout my time getting ready, I'm cognizant of how much time I have to get to the gym, juice, gratitude, etc. This makes it fun each morning attempting to get more in, and smash my time. The timer also causes me to focus 100 percent on what I'm doing right then and there. Many people multitask. When we multitask our brain function decreases by 45 percent. This is a surefire way to keep you engaged in one single activity, ensuring your success.

Intrinsic Value System

Once the habit is formed it becomes part of your overall lifestyle and, in turn, your habits transcend into your values. If you can set your standards up to this level then you've got it. Having sustainability once you cherish and value this new routine should make it next to impossible for you to fail. There will be times when you just can't make it to the gym, or go for a walk, run, jog, yoga, etc.

DO NOT beat yourself up for it. Always honor yourself for your courageous discipline and enjoy the day off. The great news is, once you manage to master your physical body, you can use this same process in all other facets of your life: spiritual, financial, relationships, communication, and so forth.

Conclusion

We can sit here and debate calories vs. carbs, or circuit training vs. long, slow running all day. But decidedly, if you don't have the mindset of the person you want to be, then you will never change. Real long-term change comes from within. Change your mind, change your body, change your life.

YOUR NEXT STEP:

I Live To Give . . .
And I give a lot of great advice on my Facebook page at

www.Facebook.com/vegetablejuicing

Go there and LIKE us to join the community of juicers and FitLifers today.

BRAND NEW BOOK FROM AUTHOR

DREW CANOLE!

On SALE Now On Amazon.com!

"Train Your Taste To Trim Your Waist:

**A Simple Method To
Love The Food That Loves You Back"**

http://trainyourtaste.com/juicingrecipes

This groundbreaking new book from Drew Canole is on sale now, exclusively at Amazon.

Revealing a simple, step-by-step method that anyone can use, to finally flip the switch and love the food that loves you back!

READ A SAMPLE ON THE NEXT PAGE

"Why does everything that's bad for me taste so good?"

Have you ever asked yourself the question above? Almost every one of us has. But consider the following.

What If healthy-food tasted delicious and fried foods made us cringe?

What if fresh steamed veggies made our mouths water?

What if a glass of freshly squeezed vegetable-juice tasted much better than a Coke or Pepsi?

And what if children actually begged for broccoli instead of cookies? (Ok, maybe *this* one is wishful thinking).

If these "what if's" were a reality for you, if you really did gravitate toward the healthiest option naturally, how difficult would it then be to lose that extra fat around your midsection?

How much easier would it be to watch weight melt off of you and finally achieve the body of your dreams, or the body of your youth, for that matter?

What if you loved the food that loves you back? What if you craved the food that makes your body run like the finely tuned machine it really is? You would never be on a "diet" and you would never be stressed out about avoiding the food you loved.

It may sound like wishful thinking, only true in fantasies. But it can be real for you.

I'm going to give you a step-by-step method to lose inches around your waist, drop fat from your body, and heal yourself from the inside out.

You will find yourself actually craving the most nourishing foods that you know you should eat—the kind of food that gives you energy and removes unwanted weight. The junky, processed foods that have a death grip on your taste buds will soon be just an occasional treat you give yourself instead of a warden keeping your weight loss plans locked up.

You are going to discover how your traitorous and unruly taste buds are literally ruining your dreams of a flat belly, six-pack abs, or just a trim, firm waistline. Like an unruly child throwing temper tantrums or an untrained dog who refuses to obey, as much as you love them they can make your life miserable until you get them under control.

Training your taste buds is the key to transforming a laborious and miserable "diet" into an effortlessly healthy and rewarding lifestyle that you enjoy.

These are the results you'll see:

Once your taste is trained, choosing the healthy option on the menu will become second nature, cooking a delicious and nurturing meal for you and your family will be welcomed, and you'll watch fat disappear easily as you gain control of your waistline, and your life.

Here is how I know this:

Do you ever follow advice given to you by strangers on the street?

I doubt it and you shouldn't. It's important for you to understand from where and from whom that advice is coming. While it's true that I am a certified nutritionist, best-selling author, and national speaker, let me tell you a story of who I really am.

When I grew up in a small, blue-collar, Michigan community, I never thought to myself: "I want to be a Transformation Specialist some day." I never thought I would help a single person transform their body, mind or health...let alone impact hundreds of thousands, perhaps millions worldwide.

However, I've accomplished this in a shorter period of time than I thought possible and we're just getting started.

But it didn't start out that way...

When I was younger, I never really thought about anyone but myself, to be completely honest. I chased instant gratification and I figured I had the rest of my life to worry about health.

I'd hit the gym once in a while but my goals were always superficial: Look good for the ladies. I didn't really care what I put into my body as long as it didn't make me sick.

But it was making me sick, from the inside out. I just didn't know it.

I was living in Tampa, Florida during the real estate boom, working in the mortgage industry and although I was making decent money, I was miserable. With stress levels at an all time high from working in a business I hated, and my belly poking out over the top of my jeans, I wondered why I was getting sick four or five times per year.

My mentor at the time pointed out everything in my life that was "out of alignment" and told me I needed to make a major change or be miserable for the rest of my life. And I was only twenty-eight years old at the time.

I wasn't proud of my career, I wasn't proud of my energy levels, I wasn't proud of my body and I felt like I was letting a lot of potential for a better life slip through my fingers.

People who know me know one thing, when I commit to something, I commit "all the way" (I encourage this habit by the way, it's highly effective).

I gave everything away (except my clothes), moved to sunny San Diego and spent a year of my life researching health and learning how to get the body I wanted. Admittedly, I have a bit of an addictive personality as well, so when I started digging into the world of fitness, I wasn't happy to just read books. I wanted to talk to the most prestigious experts who were doing cutting-edge research and getting the best results.

My one criterion, whatever health or fitness regimen I followed was: it would have to be holistically healthy for my mind, body and my soul and NATURAL. No more selling myself short just to try to get a six-pack fast...this was my life we were talking about.

The next year was filled with me weaseling my way in to talk to nationally recognized experts, doctors and fitness specialists. I went to Mexico to a healing center and to places all over California exploring every option I could find.

The results: it all came down to eating good, whole foods, exercising and cultivating a positive mindset. That's the simple explanation, not exactly rocket-science, is it?

I soon realized that the difficult portion would be to re-train myself to enjoy eating good food, working out consistently and staying positive even when the day was trying to beat me down.

But I did it (and you will too).

Along the way, I shared my progress, photos and some very rough Youtube videos on Facebook.com/thinkfeelbecome. I invited my friends to follow my progress. I'm happy to say that the progress went faster than my friends or I ever thought possible.

After only 6 months, I went from 17.2% to 5.75% body fat. And it happened naturally, without drugs, steroids or other unhealthy methods.

Side note: Something very important happens when you enlist others in your success...they join you.

Soon I had my first transformation client who offered me $3,000 to be his virtual coach, from 3,000 miles away and to help lead both him and his wife through the process that I went through. Ninety days later, they both had remarkable results.

Soon, one by one, through word of mouth, people sought me out. My knowledge was growing and with every person I taught, I learned more than they did. I began to understand what limits people, what motivates them and the diverse range of challenges we all face on the way to our health and fitness goals.

Within six months of my first client, I was now being paid $10,000 per client to create the transformation experience for them.

Certain celebrities (whose names must remain private) contacted me for transformation coaching and television producers are now pitching me talk show and infomercial ideas. For a guy who simply shared his success and strategies with those who were willing to listen, the ride has been fun and overwhelming at the same time.

But I keep my focus on my clients. Although each individual faced different challenges, I'm proud to say that 100% of them have not only reached, but often exceeded their fitness goals. That is how I know that what I'm about to teach you works.

You don't have to listen to me, but I highly encourage you to open your mind and follow my advice, especially if nothing has worked for you so far.

Chapter 2:
Abs Are Made In The Kitchen

I used to think that doing hundreds of sit ups and long, boring hours of cardio in the gym was the key to a flat stomach and sixpack abs. From crunches, to leg-lifts, to side bends, I did every imaginable exercise for years until I realized that everything was for naught unless I was eating correctly.

Perhaps you experienced the same frustration. If you're like many people, you think that as long as you work out hard, you can probably eat whatever you want. For some people (like athletes) that might be true. For others though, it's a different story. Most people don't have enough hours in the day to work off all of the calories they pour into their body every day.

Furthermore, our bodies respond much better and more quickly to food than they do to exercise. It's been said that 80% of your success is determined by your diet. (I think it's more than that). As important as both of them are, it's the food we put in our body determines the primary shape of our body.

And contrary to popular belief, all calories are not created equal. Fat calories, protein calories, and carbohydrate calories cause our body to react differently. But even more dramatic than that is the difference between whole, nourishing foods (like meats and vegetables) and processed foods (like 90% of the grocery store) in the way our body metabolizes them and uses them for fuel or for fat.

If you drove a sports car, would you put the cheapest gas in it? Some people do.

Recently I was on my way to the beach with my friend Jack. As a passenger in his beautiful BMW M5, which cost more than some people's houses, I was admiring how well it handled and how it really *is* the ultimate driving machine.

We stopped for gas and Jack went into the convenience store to grab a Big Gulp of soda and bag of chips. When he returned he filled up his tank with 93 octane gas. I looked at Jack, then at his Big Gulp, then back at Jack. I asked him, "Why do you put the most expensive gas in your tank, Jack... with gas prices so high?" His answer was exactly what I expected it to be: "Drew, when you own the 'Ultimate Driving Machine' you gotta take care of it— even if it costs a little more."

With a quick glance back at his Big Gulp, I left it at that. Jack never saw his own body as an ultimate anything, let alone the machine that he drives every day of his life. If he did, I'm positive he'd be drinking a bottle of water instead of the chemical soup he calls soda.

Jack is my friend and he doesn't really see himself as having a problem. It's not my job to preach to deaf ears. I find it much more rewarding to help those who have already decided that their lives are worth it, and who believe their bodies are the Ultimate Living Machines.